Healing in Harmony

Vital Insights into Integrative Therapy

Dr. Jyotika Sharma

Col. Surajit Debnath (Retd.)

AF658277

BookMyStory®

Healing in Harmony
Vital Insights into Integrative Therapy
Dr. Jyotika Sharma & Col. Surajit Debnath(Retd.)

Published in 2025

© Dr. Jyotika Sharma & Col. Surajit Debnath(Retd.)

© Published by

BookMyStory®

It's time you tell your story

BookMyStory
Thane, 400615, India
info@bookmystorypublishing.com
www.bookmystorypublishing.com

All rights reserved
No part of this publication may be reproduced, stored in a retrieval system, or transmitted in any form or by any means, electronic, mechanical, photocopying, recording or otherwise, without the prior permission of the author.

ISBN: 978-93-49509-93-1 [Paperback / softback]

Foreword

Healthcare today often feels rushed and transactional–a quick consultation, a prescription, and a polite "take care." But deep down, we know healing is more than that. It's about connection. It's about being seen, heard, and cared for–not just as a patient, but as a whole human being.

Healing in Harmony: Vital Insights into Integrative Therapy is a beautiful reminder of what medicine can and should be. It doesn't pit modern science against traditional wisdom; instead, it weaves them together into a tapestry of thoughtful, compassionate care.

This book invites you to slow down and reimagine what wellness means. Through clear explanations and evidence-backed insights, it brings the world of integrative health within reach–whether you're curious about mindfulness, exploring herbal remedies, or searching for a path that feels more personal and sustainable.

What I love most about this book is its inclusivity. It's for everyone—patients seeking clarity, practitioners striving for balance, and caregivers navigating the emotional terrain of supporting a loved one. Each chapter is an open hand, offering practical tools, gentle wisdom, and the reassurance that healing is not a destination but a journey.

As you turn these pages, I hope you find what so many of us are looking for—a sense of possibility, empowerment, and harmony in your own healing story.

Welcome to a world where healthcare listens, integrates, and truly heals.

Cdr (Dr) G L Sharma
Vice Chancellor,
SRM University, Gangtok,
Sikkim, India

Table of Contents

Foreword 3

Introduction: A New Way to Heal 7

Chapter 1: What Are Integrative Therapies–and Why Are They Changing Healthcare? 11

Chapter 2: The Biomedical Vs. Integrative Approach 19

Chapter 3: From "Alternative" To Integrative–How Healing Came Full Circle 29

Chapter 4: Patient-Centred Care In Action 37

Chapter 5: The Science Behind The Healing 47

Chapter 6: Creating Your Integrative Care Plan 55

Chapter 7: Integrative Therapies In Clinical Practice 63

Chapter 8: Integrative Care Across Life Stages 73

Chapter 9: Policy, Access & The Future Of Integrative Health 83

Conclusion: A Return To Wholeness 91

References & Suggested Reading 97

About The Authors 101

Introduction:
A New Way To Heal

Why This Book?

What if your doctor's visit included a conversation about your favourite meals, your stress levels, your sleep, and how often you laugh?

What if your treatment plan included both medication and meditation?

Welcome to the world of integrative health—where science meets tradition, and healing means caring for your whole self.

This book is for anyone who's ever felt that something was missing in their healthcare journey. Whether you're a patient, practitioner, caregiver, or curious soul, you're in the right place.

What Is Integrative Health?

Let's clear this up right away:

Integrative health is not about ditching modern medicine. It's about adding to it, thoughtfully and respectfully.

It combines:

- Conventional medical treatments
- Evidence-based complementary therapies
- Emotional and mental well-being
- Lifestyle choices, movement, and nutrition
- Deep listening and patient-centred care

It's not a "one-size-fits-all" approach. It's about **what works best for you**—physically, emotionally, and spiritually.

What You'll Find Inside

This isn't a medical textbook. It's a friendly guide—equal parts practical and soulful.

Each chapter offers:

- Simple language
- Clear explanations of integrative tools
- Science you can understand
- Inspiring examples from clinics and communities
- Tips to help you start your healing plan

Think of it as a roadmap—with options at every turn.

Why It Matters Now

Our world is changing fast, and so are our health needs.

- Chronic illnesses are rising
- Burnout is real
- Pills alone aren't enough
- People want care that honours their story, not just their symptoms

Integrative care isn't just "nice to have." It's urgently needed to build a healthcare system that listens, adapts, and truly heals.

Ready to Begin?

You don't need to be an expert. You don't need to "believe" in anything.

You just need curiosity–and a willingness to explore what healing might look like, beyond the usual scripts.

So, take a deep breath.
Turn the page.
And step into a story of **healing that honours all of you.**

Chapter 1:

What Are Integrative Therapies—and Why Are They Changing Healthcare?

A New Way to Heal

In today's world, where stress is constant and chronic illness is common, many people are asking:

"Is there more to healing than prescriptions and procedures?"

Yes, there is. And that "more" is called **integrative therapy**—a way of treating not just disease, but the *whole person.*

Integrative care blends the best of conventional medicine with time-tested healing practices. It doesn't replace modern science—it enhances it, weaving mind, body, and spirit into one powerful approach to health.

What Is Integrative Therapy?

Integrative therapies combine standard medical treatments with safe, evidence-informed complementary approaches, like acupuncture, meditation, herbal medicine, or yoga.

They aim to:

- Reduce side effects
- Boost emotional and mental well-being
- Manage chronic conditions
- Promote long-term health and vitality

The Core Principles

Integrative care is more than just a collection of therapies. It's a **philosophy** built on four core values:

Whole-Person Focus

You are not just a symptom. Integrative care looks at your body, emotions, environment, relationships, and sense of meaning.

Evidence-Informed

Therapies are chosen based on scientific research, expert experience, and patient preference—not guesswork.

Collaborative Partnership

The patient becomes a **partner** in the healing process, actively involved in decision-making.

Least Invasive First

Care begins with gentle, low-risk options—and escalates only when needed.

The Toolkit: Types of Integrative Therapies

1. Mind-Body Practices

- Meditation
- Breathwork
- Yoga, Tai Chi, Qigong
- Guided imagery

Balances the nervous system and reduces stress.

2. Manual and Movement Therapies

- Massage therapy
- Chiropractic care
- Craniosacral therapy

Improves circulation, mobility, and muscle release.

3. Nutritional & Herbal Approaches

- Anti-inflammatory diets
- Herbal remedies (e.g., turmeric, ashwagandha)
- Supplements (e.g., vitamin D, omega-3)

Supports the immune system, energy, and healing.

4. Energy-Based Therapies

- Reiki
- Healing Touch
- Chakra balancing

Promotes calm and pain relief; many patients report emotional clarity.

5. Traditional Systems of Medicine

- **Ayurveda (India)**
- **Traditional Chinese Medicine (TCM)**
- **Unani and Indigenous practices**

Based on centuries of wisdom, customised to body type and constitution.

Wait, Is This the Same as "Alternative Medicine"?

Not exactly.

Alternative Medicine	Integrative Medicine
Replaces conventional care	Works alongside it
Often used instead of drugs.	Combines the best of both
Can risk missing vital treatments	Supports safe, ethical collaboration

A cancer patient might get chemotherapy (conventional) and acupuncture (integrative)—both together in one care plan.

Backed by Science

Many integrative practices are supported by strong research:

- **Mindfulness:** reduces anxiety and depression
- **Acupuncture:** relieves migraines and arthritis pain
- **Yoga:** improves PTSD, back pain, and sleep
- **Nutrition:** reduces inflammation and supports heart health

Around the Globe

In many parts of the world, integrative medicine is mainstream.

- **India:** Ayurveda and yoga in public health
- **China:** TCM integrated with hospitals
- **Germany/Switzerland:** Homoeopathy covered by insurance
- **Brazil:** Herbal medicine and spiritual healing in clinics

Healing doesn't look the same everywhere—and that's a strength.

Why People Choose Integrative Care

Millions of people are embracing integrative options. Why?

- To feel empowered
- To avoid medication side effects

- To explore natural or holistic solutions
- To support chronic disease management
- To align care with spiritual or cultural values
- Studies show higher satisfaction and better quality of life among integrative care users.

Common Myths—Debunked

Myth	**Reality**
"It's anti-science."	Many therapies are evidence-based.
"Only for wealthy people."	Digital tools and group care make it accessible.
"It's all spiritual fluff."	It treats physical symptoms too, with real tools.

Ethics and Safety First

Ethical integrative care is:

- Safe - avoids risky detoxes or false cures
- Transparent - about credentials and evidence
- **Patient-centred** - honours your values and choices
- **Collaborative** - works with other healthcare providers

It's not about magic—it's about mindful, meaningful care.

Looking Ahead

Integrative care is not a trend—it's a shift in how we understand health. The future includes:

- Better insurance coverage
- More research into ancient practices
- Greater medical training in holistic care
- Cultural healing is being honoured and included

The world is rediscovering the wisdom of balance.

Final Words: A More Human Approach

Integrative therapy is about more than health—it's about healing.

It reminds us that we are more than our test results. We are people with stories, beliefs, families, fears, and hope.

Whether you're a patient seeking answers or a provider seeking more meaning in care, integrative therapy opens the door to something deeper, more connected, and more complete.

Chapter 2:
The Biomedical Vs. Integrative Approach

Two Views of Health: Head-to-Head

Healthcare today often feels like a tug of war between two models:

- The **biomedical model**, which dominates hospitals and clinics
- The **integrative model**, which is growing in popularity worldwide

Both aim to help us heal, but they go about it in very different ways.

Let's explore the contrast. Think of this as a friendly match-up, not a battle.

The Biomedical Model: Precision, Science, and Structure

The **biomedical model** focuses on:

- **Physical causes** of disease (like bacteria, genetics, trauma)
- **Diagnosis and treatment** using labs, scans, and drugs
- **Specialisation**—doctors for every organ and function
- **Short-term fixes**—treat the illness, not always the whole person

It'*s based on* ***objectivity,*** *data, and reproducibility. And it has saved countless lives.*

Strengths:

- Emergency and acute care
- Infections, injuries, surgeries
- Diagnostic accuracy
- Evidence-based treatment

Limits:

- Less focus on prevention or emotional health
- May overlook lifestyle, stress, or personal history
- Patients often feel like "cases," not people

The Integrative Model: Healing the Whole Person

The **integrative model** takes a broader lens. It views health as a balance of body, mind, and environment, rather than just the absence of disease.

It combines the best of modern medicine with:

- Mind-body practices
- Nutrition and lifestyle
- Emotional and spiritual care
- Traditional healing systems

The patient is a ***partner,*** *not a passive recipient. Treatment plans are often co-created.*

Strengths:

- Holistic, person-centred care
- Emphasis on prevention and wellness
- Gentle, low-risk interventions
- Builds trust and long-term resilience

Limits:

- Sometimes lacks funding and standardisation
- Not all practices are fully evidence-backed (yet)
- May not be suited for acute crises

Quick Comparison: Biomedical vs. Integrative

Feature	Biomedical Model	Integrative Model
Focus	Disease treatment	Whole-person healing
Approach	Reactive	Proactive + preventive
Therapies	Drugs, surgery	Nutrition, yoga, herbs, counselling
Care style	Doctor-driven	Patient-partnered
Goal	Cure illness	Improve quality of life
Time spent	Often brief	Usually longer, more personal

The Mind Matters Too

Biomedical care excels in precision, but often neglects **how we feel**, think, and cope.

Science now shows the **mind-body connection** is real:

- Stress raises inflammation
- Trauma affects gut health
- Emotions impact immunity

Integrative care *uses this knowledge* through meditation, breathwork, therapy, and compassionate listening.

Example: A patient with Irritable Bowel Syndrome (IBS) may get medication *and* mindfulness-based stress reduction. That's integrative thinking.

Human Connection Is Healing

Patients often say what helped them most wasn't a pill—it was **being heard.** Integrative care honours the **relationship** between practitioner and patient.

It encourages:

- Storytelling
- Shared decision-making
- Respect for personal beliefs
- Seeing the patient as a person, not just a diagnosis

One patient put it this way:

"My integrative doctor didn't just ask about my symptoms. She asked how I was doing."

What About the Science?

Biomedical care leans on:

- Randomised controlled trials (RCTs)
- Measurable biomarkers
- Population-level data

Integrative care uses:

- RCTs **and** qualitative studies (e.g., how people feel)
- Real-world patient outcomes
- Personalised data and preferences

Today, leading journals publish research on yoga for back pain, acupuncture for migraines, and mindfulness for anxiety.

The two worlds are converging—and that's good news.

Training and Philosophy

Aspect	Biomedical Education	Integrative Training
Duration	5–10 years	Often shorter (but evolving)
Emphasis	Anatomy, pharmacology, pathology	Holism, communication, nutrition
Patient Role	Passive recipient	Active participant
View of Health	Absence of disease	State of complete well-being

Note: Many integrative providers are also MDs, nurses, or psychologists. The best care blends the two.

A Tale of Two Visits

Biomedical Visit Example

- 15-minute consultation
- Focus: blood pressure, cholesterol
- Prescription given
- Follow-up in 6 months

Integrative Visit Example

- 45-minute session
- Discussion of stress, sleep, diet, and emotions
- Plan includes meditation, magnesium, and a walking routine
- Regular follow-up and adjustments

Both are valuable—just very different in style and depth.

Why the Shift?

People are craving more meaningful, personalised care. They want answers that don't just come in a bottle.

The rise in chronic diseases, mental health struggles, and burnout has led to:

- More **lifestyle diseases** like diabetes and obesity
- More **mental-emotional fatigue**
- More **information-savvy patients** seeking options

Integrative care answers that call, without throwing out the advances of modern medicine.

Can They Work Together?

Absolutely.

The **ideal future** blends the best of both:

Biomedical care for:

- Heart attacks
- Infections
- Surgery
- Diagnostics

Integrative care for:

- Stress-related illness
- Autoimmune and chronic conditions
- Mental wellness
- Prevention and recovery

A cardiologist might treat heart disease and recommend stress reduction. That's modern integrative care.

Building the Best of Both Worlds

If you're a healthcare provider, here's how to bridge the models:

1. Listen deeply—go beyond symptoms.
2. Use evidence-based complementary therapies.
3. Refer and collaborate with integrative practitioners.
4. Honour patient values and cultural traditions.
5. Educate and empower—patients deserve options.

Integrative care doesn't ask you to abandon science—it asks you to **humanise** it.

Final Thoughts: It's Not Either/Or. It's Both.

The future of healthcare **is not a battle between models.** It's a blending–a collaboration.

The biomedical model gave us vaccines, surgical miracles, and life-saving drugs.

The **integrative model** brings meaning, connection, and self-care into the picture.

Together, they offer a path to **health that heals more than just the body.**

Chapter 3:

From "Alternative" To Integrative—How Healing Came Full Circle

What's in a Name?

Once upon a time, therapies like acupuncture, herbal medicine, and meditation were labelled "alternative." That word often made them sound fringe, unscientific, or even suspect.

But times have changed.

What we now call **integrative health** has come a long way—from the outskirts of medicine to a growing presence in hospitals, clinics, and research centres.

This chapter examines how Complementary and Alternative Medicine (CAM) evolved into Integrative Health, and why this shift is significant for patients, providers, and the future of healing.

A Brief History of Healing

Long before hospitals and white coats, people healed with herbs, touch, breath, and rituals. Across cultures–from Ayurveda in India to Traditional Chinese Medicine–health was seen as balance.

But the 20th century brought a revolution in science and technology. The **biomedical model** took centre stage, and older practices were often dismissed as unscientific.

Still, people continued to seek them, especially when conventional care didn't meet all their needs.

Defining the Terms

Term	What It Means
Alternative Medicine	Used *instead of* conventional medicine
Complementary Medicine	Used *alongside* conventional treatment
CAM (Complementary & Alternative Medicine)	Umbrella term for both
Integrative Health	Combines safe, evidence-informed CAM with conventional care in a coordinated way

"Alternative" implies a choice between one or the other. "Integrative" brings the best of both together.

Why the Clamour?

1. Rising Demand

Patients began asking for more holistic options:

- "Can I manage this without so many pills?"
- "What can I do for the stress behind my symptoms?"
- "How can I take control of my health?"

2. Scientific Interest

Researchers started to study yoga, acupuncture, meditation, and herbal remedies. Evidence grew, especially for conditions like:

- Chronic pain
- Anxiety and depression
- Insomnia
- IBS and migraines

3. Mainstream Integration

Hospitals and clinics began offering:

- Acupuncture for cancer patients
- Reiki in pre-op areas
- Mindfulness training for staff
- Diet and lifestyle programs for diabetes

Changing Mindsets: From "Fixing" to "Supporting"

The old way: "You're broken; let's fix you."

The integrative way: "You're a whole person; let's support your healing."

This new approach acknowledges:

- The mind-body connection
- The value of nutrition, movement, and rest
- The role of relationships and environment
- The importance of emotional and spiritual health

Why Language Matters

Let's face it—words shape perception.

- "**Alternative**" can sound rebellious or risky
- "**Complementary**" sounds supportive, but still secondary
- "**Integrative**" is about teamwork, collaboration, and mutual respect

For patients, this signals safety and trust.

For doctors, it means science and standards matter.

For systems, it opens doors to culturally inclusive care.

CAM to Integrative: A Side-by-Side Look

CAM	Integrative Health
Often self-guided	Coordinated with the healthcare team
Viewed as "optional"	Increasingly evidence-informed
Focused on therapy	Focused on whole-person care
Variable training	Standardizing education
Limited insurance coverage	Growing inclusion in public/private plans

Research & Recognition

Integrative health isn't "alternative" anymore–**it's studied, regulated, and respected.**

Examples of high-quality evidence:

- **MBSR (Mindfulness-Based Stress Reduction):** Reduces anxiety, chronic pain, PTSD
- **Acupuncture:** Effective for migraines, osteoarthritis, chemotherapy side effects
- **Yoga and Tai Chi:** Improve balance, joint pain, sleep, and mental health
- **Nutrition-based interventions:** Lower blood sugar, blood pressure, and inflammation

Peer-reviewed journals now regularly publish on integrative practices.

Global Perspective

- **India:** AYUSH ministry supports Ayurveda, Yoga, Unani, Siddha, and Homoeopathy
- **China:** TCM is integrated into hospitals and insurance
- **Germany:** Herbal medicine and homoeopathy covered by public plans
- **Brazil:** National Policy for Integrative and Complementary Practices **(PNPIC)**

Around the world, integration is not a fringe movement–it's national policy.

What Patients Say

"My doctor prescribed meditation, not just pills. I felt like a human, not a machine."

"Adding acupuncture helped my chemo side effects more than I expected."

"The integrative team looked at my whole life, not just my cholesterol."

These stories reflect what the research confirms: **people want healing, not just treatment.**

What's Next?

- Medical education now includes integrative topics
- Insurance coverage is expanding

- Technology is connecting patients to apps, coaches, and tele-wellness
- Community-based integrative care is helping reduce costs and improve outcomes

The future is not about choosing one system over the other. It's about **weaving them together.**

Summary Snapshot

Then (CAM)	Now (Integrative Health)
Fringe or DIY	Integrated with hospitals
Limited research	Evidence-supported
Often unregulated	Professional standards growing
Optional add-on	The core part of wellness strategies
"Either/or" mindset	"Both/and" collaboration

Final Thoughts: Healing That Respects the Whole Person

The journey from CAM to Integrative Health is a story of inclusion, openness, and evolution.

We no longer have to choose between ancient wisdom and modern science.

We can choose both.

We can build systems that treat bodies and lives.

We can offer healing that is respectful, inclusive, and complete.

Chapter 4: Patient-Centred Care In Action

What If Healthcare Put People First?

Imagine walking into a clinic where your doctor doesn't just ask, "What's wrong with you?" but rather,

"What matters to you?"

That's the heart of **patient-centred care**–a shift from treating diseases to truly caring for people.

In integrative health, this isn't just a buzzword. It's the foundation.

What Is Patient-Centred Care?

Patient-centred care means putting the patient–not the disease–at the centre of every healthcare decision.

Instead of being told what to do, patients are:

- Listened to
- Respected
- Empowered to co-create their care plan
- Seen as whole people, not just diagnoses

It's about forming a partnership where your goals, beliefs, and lifestyle shape your healing journey.

The Old Way vs. The Integrative Way

Conventional Care	Patient-Centred Care
"Doctor knows best"	"Let's decide together"
10-minute rushed visits	Time to talk and listen
Focus on the disease.	Focus on the whole person.
Standardized treatments	Personalised, flexible plans
Medical hierarchy	Equal, collaborative relationships

This approach doesn't reject science. It simply honours the human behind the symptoms.

Real Story: Rani's Journey

Rani, 45, suffered from chronic migraines. She had tried multiple medications with little relief and many side effects.

At an integrative clinic, things changed. Instead of another pill, she was asked:

- "What's your daily routine like?"
- "When did the headaches begin?"
- "What helps you relax?"

Her new care plan included:

- Acupuncture twice a month
- Magnesium-rich diet
- Breathing exercises before bed
- Reducing screen time in the evening

Within 8 weeks, her migraines were less frequent, and she felt hopeful for the first time.

Listening Is a Medical Tool

In traditional care, doctors may interrupt patients within seconds. In integrative settings, the goal is to **listen.**

Why? Because:

- Symptoms often connect to lifestyle, stress, or trauma
- People feel more engaged when they're heard
- Stories can reveal patterns that tests can't

Healing begins when patients feel safe, seen, and heard.

The Patient as a Partner

A key shift in integrative health is seeing the **patient as a partner**, not a passive receiver.

That means:

- Asking about values, fears, and goals
- Co-creating care plans
- Encouraging questions and feedback
- Respecting cultural preferences and beliefs

The result? Better outcomes—and happier, more empowered patients.

Personalisation in Practice

One size does not fit all.

Here's how personalisation might look:

Symptom	Conventional Approach	Integrative Approach
High blood pressure	Medication	Medication + diet + stress reduction
Insomnia	Sleep aids	Sleep hygiene + guided imagery + herbal support
Chronic pain	Painkillers	Movement therapy + acupuncture + mindset work
Depression	Antidepressants	Talk therapy + mindfulness + nutrition

Like painting a portrait, integrative care considers each individual's unique canvas.

A Toolkit for Whole-Person Healing

In a patient-centred model, treatment isn't just pills and procedures. It might include:

- **Lifestyle coaching**
- **Movement practices** like yoga or tai chi
- **Emotional support,** like counselling or art therapy
- **Nutrition guidance** tailored to your needs
- **Energy healing** for grounding and relief
- **Mind-body techniques** for stress management

It's not about choosing *one* thing–it's about layering small, supportive tools to create meaningful change.

Why It Works

Research shows that **patient-centred integrative** care can lead to:

- Better symptom control
- Lower medication use
- Higher patient satisfaction
- Fewer hospital visits
- Improved mental health

People feel **motivated** when they are part of the process, not just subjects in a system.

What Providers Can Learn

Even providers trained in the biomedical model can shift their approach by:

- Asking open-ended questions
- Practising active listening
- Giving space for emotion
- Acknowledging the mind-body connection
- Including patients in decisions

The best medicine is not always found in a bottle. Sometimes it's in a conversation.

Cultural Sensitivity Matters

True patient-centred care is also **culturally respectful.**

That means:

- Honouring traditional beliefs or healing rituals
- Adapting care plans to fit family dynamics
- Being aware of language, gender roles, or religious needs
- Involving community healers or spiritual leaders if helpful

Healing is deeply personal—and often, deeply cultural.

Real Story: Abhay's Path to Healing

Abhay, a 60-year-old man with Type 2 diabetes, didn't trust doctors.

At his first visit to an integrative centre, the provider asked:

"What do you believe caused your illness?"

Abhay said it was years of grief and stress. The provider didn't dismiss it. Instead, they explored both medical and emotional paths.

His care included:

- Blood sugar monitoring
- A walking group
- Talking to a counsellor about grief
- Learning to cook with traditional spices and oils

For Abhay, healing came through **connection**, not just medication.

Follow-Up and Flexibility

Integrative care is not a "one-and-done" visit. It involves:

- Regular check-ins
- Adjusting treatments based on progress
- Encouraging self-reflection
- Celebrating small wins

Healing takes time, and a flexible, compassionate plan supports that journey.

The Digital Bridge

Patient-centred care is going virtual too:

- Health apps for mindfulness or medication tracking
- Telehealth visits with integrative specialists
- Online support communities
- Wearables to track sleep, stress, and activity

When used wisely, tech becomes a tool for empowerment, not a barrier.

Summary Snapshot

Element	Description
Listening	Time and space for the patient's story
Empathy	Meeting people where they are
Collaboration	Shared decision-making
Cultural respect	Honour values, language, and traditions
Personalization	No cookie-cutter treatment plans
Ongoing support	Flexibility and follow-up matter

Final Thoughts: Care That Feels Like Care

True healing happens when people feel heard, respected, and involved in their care. That's what **patient-centred integrative care offers.**

It's not about choosing between tradition and science–it's

about choosing compassion, connection, and collaboration.

Whether you're a patient or a provider, this model reminds us of something deeply human:

Healing is not just about what we do–it's about how we show up for each other.

Chapter 5: The Science Behind The Healing

"Is There Proof?"

That's one of the first questions people ask about integrative therapies:

"Sounds interesting, but... is there evidence it works?"

Fair question. And the short answer? **Yes–plenty.**

Over the past two decades, science has been catching up with what many cultures have known for centuries: that healing is more than medicine alone. Let's take a closer look.

What Does "Evidence-Based" Really Mean?

When we say a therapy is evidence-based, it means there's reliable research–often clinical trials or long-term studies–showing it works for certain conditions.

But in integrative health, evidence comes in many forms:

- Clinical trials (RCTs)
- Observational studies
- Patient-reported outcomes
- Longstanding use in traditional systems

Good care = Science + Experience + What works for the individual

Mind-Body Practices: Healing Through Awareness

These therapies show how thoughts, emotions, and physical health are linked:

Mindfulness Meditation

- **What it helps:** anxiety, depression, pain, and blood pressure
- **The science:** Research shows changes in brain structure, reduced cortisol levels, and improved focus after 8 weeks of practice
- **Popular program:** MBSR (Mindfulness-Based Stress Reduction)

Yoga & Tai Chi

- **What they help:** arthritis, PTSD, back pain, balance issues
- **The science:** Improve strength, flexibility, mood, and sleep

Fun fact: Yoga has been studied in over 1,000 peer-reviewed articles!

Acupuncture: Needles That Nurture

Used for thousands of years in Chinese medicine, acupuncture is now mainstream in many hospitals.

The evidence:

- Reduces chronic pain (back, neck, knees)
- Helps with migraine, tension headaches
- Eases chemotherapy-related nausea
- May assist in fertility and menopausal symptoms

Studies show acupuncture activates the nervous system, releases endorphins, and improves blood flow.

Nutrition as Medicine

Food isn't just fuel–it's one of our most powerful healing tools.

What the research shows:

- **Mediterranean Diet:** Lowers risk of heart disease, stroke, and Alzheimer's
- **Plant-based diets:** Help manage diabetes and reduce inflammation
- **Anti-inflammatory foods:** Like turmeric, ginger, leafy greens–linked to better mood and immune support

In integrative care, food becomes part of the prescription, not just an afterthought.

Herbal and Natural Therapies

Many plants have potent health benefits. But which ones are supported by science?

Herb	What It's Used For	Evidence Highlights
Ashwagandha	Stress, anxiety	Shown to reduce cortisol and improve sleep
Turmeric (Curcumin)	Inflammation, joint pain	Strong anti-inflammatory and antioxidant
Peppermint oil	IBS, digestion	Effective for bloating and cramping
Lavender	Anxiety, sleep	Helps with relaxation and insomnia

Note: Always check for quality, dosage, and drug interactions.

Creative Therapies: Healing Through Expression

Integrative care often uses **art, music, and movement** to support emotional healing.

The science:

- **Art therapy:** Helps trauma survivors express and process feelings
- **Music therapy:** Eases anxiety in patients with cancer or dementia

- **Dance/movement therapy:** Improves motor skills, especially in Parkinson's patients

It's not about being "good" at art–it's about tapping into feelings that words can't always reach.

Psychoneuroimmunology: Mind-Body Medicine in Action

Big word, simple idea:

Your **mind, nervous system, and immune system** talk to each other constantly.

Stress, for example, raises inflammation. Chronic worry affects digestion and immunity.

Studies show:

- Meditation improves immune markers
- Social support reduces hospital stays
- Gratitude practice lowers heart disease risk

Healing isn't just physical. Emotions matter–a lot.

Who's Doing the Research?

You might be surprised by the prestigious institutions involved in integrative health research:

- **Harvard Osher Centre for Integrative Medicine**
- **University of California, San Francisco (UCSF)**

- **MD Anderson Cancer Centre**
- **Cleveland Clinic's Centre for Functional Medicine**
- **National Centre for Complementary and Integrative Health (NCCIH)**

They're not studying "woo-woo." They're studying what works—carefully, rigorously, and respectfully.

What About Safety?

Like any treatment, integrative therapies must be used responsibly.

What to look for:

- Certified practitioners
- Evidence-based therapies
- Communication with your doctor
- Awareness of herb-drug interactions

Not every "natural" product is safe. But with proper guidance, many integrative therapies are low-risk and high-reward.

Real Patient Voices

"I tried acupuncture for migraines. I was sceptical—but it changed my life."

"Meditation helped me more than any pill ever did for my anxiety."

"Working with a health coach finally made me feel in control of my diabetes."

These aren't just testimonials–they reflect what thousands of patients report across clinical studies.

What Doctors Are Saying

"I used to dismiss integrative medicine. Now I use it daily in my practice."

"Patients don't just want a prescription. They want to be heard."

"We're seeing better outcomes when we treat the whole person."

Many conventional doctors are embracing integrative practices not out of trendiness, but because they see results.

Summary Snapshot: Therapies Backed by Research

Therapy	Supported For
Mindfulness	Stress, pain, anxiety, and Post-Traumatic Stress Disorder (PTSD)
Yoga	Back pain, depression, and balance
Acupuncture	Migraines, arthritis, and nausea
Nutrition	Heart health, diabetes, and inflammation
Herbal medicine	Anxiety, IBS, joint health
Music/art therapy	Dementia, trauma, anxiety

Final Thoughts: The Science of Wholeness

Science is no longer a barrier to integrative health–it's a bridge.

We now know that:

- Thoughts can change our biology
- Emotions can influence recovery
- Food and movement are medicine
- Nature, music, and stillness–all play a role in healing

Evidence-based integrative care is not wishful thinking. It's **compassion backed by research.**

In the end, healing is both a science and an art.

Chapter 6:

Creating Your Integrative Care Plan

Healing That's Truly Yours

If you've made it this far, you've probably realised something important:

Healing isn't one-size-fits-all.

Your body, your story, your goals—they're all unique. So your care plan should be, too.

This chapter walks you through how to build a **personalised integrative care plan**—one that fits your life, your values, and your health goals.

Where Do You Begin?

Creating an integrative plan doesn't mean adding 10 new things to your day. It starts with three simple steps:

1. Know yourself
2. Set clear goals
3. Choose gentle, doable actions

Let's break it down.

Step 1: Get Curious About You

Before making changes, pause and reflect:

- What are your top 1–2 health concerns?
- What's been missing from your current care?
- What gives you energy, and what drains you?
- What has helped you feel better in the past?

Take a few minutes to write your answers. They will shape your plan.

Step 2: Define What "Better" Looks Like

Be specific. Instead of "I want to be healthy," try:

- "I want to sleep through the night"
- "I want to feel calmer in stressful moments"
- "I want fewer migraines each month"
- "I want to feel more in control of my blood sugar"

Ask yourself:

"How will I know if this is working?"

Your goals guide everything that follows.

Step 3: Choose Your Tools

Integrative care uses many tools—from science-backed medicine to ancient healing arts. You don't need them all. Pick what fits you best.

Here's a menu to build from:

Mind-Body Practices

Support emotional balance, focus, and stress relief.

Practice	Try If You Want To...
Mindfulness meditation	Reduce anxiety or reactivity.
Deep breathing	Calm your nervous system.
Yoga or tai chi	Improve flexibility and inner peace.
Guided imagery	Ease pain or fall asleep more easily

Nutrition and Supplements

Nourish your body and address inflammation.

Focus Area	Simple Actions
Anti-inflammatory eating	Add more colourful veggies, healthy fats.
Blood sugar balance	Eat whole grains, avoid sugary drinks.
Gut health	Include fermented foods, fibre.
Supplements	Start with vitamin D, magnesium (if needed)

Movement and Physical Therapies

Support energy, strength, and pain relief.

Practice	Benefits
Walking daily	Boosts heart health and mood
Stretching	Reduces tension and stiffness
Massage or chiropractic	Eases musculoskeletal pain
Dance or expressive movement	Uplifts emotions and body connection

Herbal and Natural Therapies

Gentle support from nature.

Herb	May Help With
Ashwagandha	Stress, fatigue
Chamomile	Sleep, digestion
Turmeric	Inflammation, joint pain
Peppermint	Headaches, IBS

Always check for interactions if on medications.

Emotional and Spiritual Care

Help you feel grounded, whole, and seen.

Tool	How It Helps
Journaling	Clarifies thoughts and feelings
Talk therapy	Builds resilience and insight
Nature time	Reduces mental overload
Prayer or ritual	Provides comfort and connection

Sample Care Plan: Meet Ananya

Ananya, 38, struggles with anxiety and poor sleep. She works long hours, skips meals, and rarely relaxes. Her integrative plan:

- **Mind-body:** 5 minutes of breathwork before bed
- **Nutrition:** No caffeine after 2 pm, protein at every meal
- **Movement:** Gentle yoga 2x/week
- **Emotional:** Evening journaling to "download" her thoughts
- **Sleep:** Magnesium supplement + screen-free wind-down at 9:30 pm

She started small and built momentum week by week.

Try This: Weekly Integrative Planner

Day	Mind-Body	Nutrition	Movement	Sleep/ Recovery	Notes
Mon	3-min breathwork	Veggie-rich lunch	20-min walk	Off screen by 9 pm	Felt focused
Tue	Gratitude journaling	Herbal tea	Yoga class	Lights out at 10 pm	Slept well
...	...	...	...	...	...

Use this to stay accountable and reflect on what's helping.

Adjust as You Go

Plans aren't permanent. Healing is dynamic.

Each week, ask:

- What felt good?
- What felt like a chore?
- What's one thing I want to change or try next?

Progress isn't always linear. Small shifts lead to big results over time.

Keep It Real: 5 Golden Rules

- **Start small** - One change at a time beats overwhelm.
- **Be consistent** - A little each day is better than a lot once a month.
- **Track progress** - Even short journal entries help.
- **Ask for help** - Coaches, providers, and peers make it easier.
- **Be kind to yourself** - Healing is a journey, not a performance.

Who Helps You Build the Plan?

You don't have to do it alone. Consider working with:

- **Integrative physicians** - blend conventional and complementary care

- **Health coaches** - help with behaviour change and habit tracking
- **Ayurvedic or TCM practitioners** - for body-type-based guidance
- **Therapists or counsellors** - to support emotional growth
- **Nutritionists** - for personalised food plans
- **Physical therapists or yoga teachers** - to ease pain and improve strength

Good integrative care is always **collaborative**, never top-down.

Real Voices

"Tracking my breath and sleep showed me how wired I was. Just 5 minutes of stillness a day changed everything." – Neeraj, 42

"My integrative plan felt like it was made for me. Not just my illness—me." – Mira, 56

"Small shifts. Huge difference." – Abhijit, 60

What to Avoid

Here's what not to include in your plan:

- Fad diets or extreme cleanses
- Expensive supplements without evidence
- Providers who don't listen

- Anything that feels forced or unsafe
- If it's not respectful, balanced, and aligned with your values, it doesn't belong in your care plan.

Summary Snapshot

Element	Why It Matters
Clear goals	Keeps your care focused
Personal reflection	Builds self-awareness
Mind-body tools	Calms and centres you.
Nutrition & movement	Fuel and flow for healing
Gentle tracking	Helps measure progress
Trusted providers	Support and guide you

Final Thoughts: Your Plan, Your Power

Creating an integrative care plan is an act of self-respect.

It says:

"I believe in my body's wisdom. I believe in healing that honours the whole of me."

You don't need to be perfect. You just need to be present.

Start small. Stay curious. Keep listening to your body, your mind, and your intuition.

The healing path is yours to walk. And every step counts.

Chapter 7:
Integrative Therapies In Clinical Practice

A New Kind of Healing Room

Walk into a growing number of hospitals today, and you might hear something unexpected:

- The soft rhythm of a singing bowl
- A patient practising guided breathing before surgery
- A nurse offering Reiki after chemotherapy

This isn't a spa–it's a **modern hospital** embracing **integrative therapies** alongside conventional care.

This chapter explores how integrative medicine is being practised in real clinical settings, blending the best of science and tradition to treat the whole person.

A Healing Partnership

In integrative healthcare, **patients aren't passive.** They're partners in their care.

And hospitals, once focused only on curing disease, are evolving into **centres for healing**–physically, emotionally, and even spiritually.

"We're no longer just treating the illness. We're treating the human experience of illness."

– Dr Leena, Oncologist

Dr Asha, an internal medicine physician in Delhi, shares: "I used to roll my eyes at herbal remedies. However, when patients continued to ask, I began researching. Now I refer them to a licensed Ayurvedic practitioner when appropriate. We collaborate. The outcomes are better, and patients feel heard."

Her shift mirrors a wider one in medicine: from control to **collaboration.**

Why the Shift?

Three key forces are driving this transformation:

1. **Patient demand:** More people want care that respects their lifestyle, values, and beliefs.

2. **Chronic illness:** Conditions like diabetes, depression, and autoimmune disorders benefit from holistic approaches.
3. **Research:** Studies now confirm the benefits of yoga, acupuncture, nutrition, and mind-body therapies.

Healing is no longer confined to prescriptions and procedures. It's becoming **collaborative, creative, and compassionate.**

What Integrative Therapies Are Being Used?

Here are some popular therapies hospitals and clinics are weaving into their care:

Therapy	Common Uses in Clinics
Acupuncture	Pain, nausea, and recovery support
Massage therapy	Stress relief, muscle tension, post-op comfort
Yoga & movement therapy	Chronic pain, mental health, and balance
Mindfulness & meditation	Anxiety, trauma, and insomnia
Nutrition counselling	Heart disease, diabetes, and cancer recovery
Art & music therapy	Emotional expression, dementia, grief support
Energy healing (Reiki, Healing Touch)	Relaxation, pre-surgery calm

Real-Life Settings Using Integrative Therapies

Cancer Care Centres

Hospitals like MD Anderson and Tata Memorial offer:

- Yoga classes for fatigue
- Acupuncture for nausea
- Nutrition support for immune strength
- Counselling for grief and hope

Patients report less anxiety, better sleep, and feeling more like themselves during treatment.

Cardiac & Stroke Recovery Units

Programs combine:

- Breathing exercises to lower blood pressure
- Tai chi for gentle movement
- Diet changes to reduce cholesterol
- Group support for lifestyle changes

These additions improve outcomes and help prevent re-hospitalisations.

Mental Health Clinics

Here, integrative therapies are reshaping recovery:

- Art therapy to unlock trauma
- Mindfulness for depression and anxiety

- Nature-based therapy to soothe the nervous system
- Group yoga or expressive movement for empowerment

Patients feel less alone and more capable of healing.

What Clinicians Say

"Acupuncture has become part of our pain management strategy. It helps reduce reliance on opioids." – Dr Raj, Orthopaedic Surgeon.

"I teach my patients a breathing practice before surgery. It's simple, quick, and incredibly calming." – Nurse Deepika.

"Integrative medicine lets me treat more than symptoms. It lets me treat stories." – Dr Neha, Family Physician.

The Integrative Team: Who's Involved?

An integrative approach often includes:

Role	Contribution
Medical doctor (MD)	Diagnoses, leads care, and manages safety
Nurse practitioner	Daily support, coordination
Yoga/mind-body therapist	Teaches practices to regulate stress
Nutritionist	Designs food-based healing strategies.
Licensed acupuncturist	Relieves pain, stress, and side effects

Counsellor/psychologist	Supports emotional resilience
Coach or patient navigator	Guides lifestyle changes and goal-setting

Together, they **co-create a plan** with the patient's voice at the centre.

What an Integrative Visit Looks Like

Here's how an integrative consultation might unfold:

1. **Extended time** - Visits often last 45–60 minutes
2. **Deep listening** - The provider asks about your life, not just your illness
3. **Goal setting** - You talk about *what healing means* to you
4. **Personalised plan** - A combination of medical and holistic strategies
5. **Follow-up** - Plans evolve based on your feedback and progress

"It felt like they saw me, not just my lab results." — Patient testimonial

Integration, Not Substitution

Integrative therapies don't replace necessary medical treatment. They **enhance** it.

For example:

- A cancer patient may take chemo **and** practice restorative yoga
- A diabetic may use insulin **and** follow a personalised nutrition plan
- A person with depression may take medication **and** learn mindfulness

The goal is not *either/or*–it's *both/and.*

The Evidence Behind the Integration

Hospitals embrace integrative care not out of trendiness, but because it works.

What research shows:

- Mindfulness reduces hospital readmissions in cardiac patients
- Acupuncture lowers chronic back pain in clinical trials
- Nutrition counselling improves blood sugar control
- Yoga improves flexibility and reduces anxiety in cancer survivors
- Music therapy reduces agitation in dementia patients

These aren't opinions–they're data-backed decisions.

Challenges and Opportunities

What's working:

- Growing demand
- Expanding research
- Patient satisfaction through the roof

What needs improvement:

- Insurance coverage
- Access in rural or low-resource settings
- Consistent training standards for practitioners

The future depends on **policy, education, and advocacy** to make integrative care accessible to all.

Real Story: Healing Beyond the Prescription

Mohan, 58, came to a cardiac centre after a minor heart attack.

Instead of just being sent home with meds, he was offered:

- A dietitian to rework his meals
- Weekly group yoga
- A stress management coach
- Regular follow-ups with his doctor

Six months later, Mohan's cholesterol dropped, his stress eased, and he felt in charge of his health.

"They didn't just treat my heart. They taught me how to live better."

Summary Snapshot

Element	What Makes It Integrative
Team approach	Doctors + complementary practitioners
Whole-person focus	Physical, emotional, social, and spiritual care
Flexible tools	From pills to Pranayam
Personalized plans	Your goals, your values, your pace
Evidence-based	Grounded in research
Empowered patients	You're part of every decision.

Final Thoughts: Healing in Real Time

Integrative therapies aren't just ideas on paper. They're happening in real clinics, with real people, making real progress.

And they remind us that healthcare can be more than functional. It can be **deeply human.**

Whether you're a patient, practitioner, or policymaker, the message is clear:

When we care for the whole person, everyone heals bet.

Chapter 8:
Integrative Care Across Life Stages

Health for Every Chapter of Life

From the first breath to the final goodbye, we go through many phases—and so does our health.

What if care changed with us? What if it honoured each season of life, not just the symptoms?

That's the beauty of **integrative care.** It's not a one-time fix. It's a lifelong partnership that adapts to who you are and where you are in life.

Early Childhood: Building a Foundation

Children are naturally resilient, but they also need support to thrive, especially with rising cases of allergies, attention issues, and anxiety.

Integrative tools for kids:

- **Massage and touch therapy:** Soothes colic, supports bonding
- **Mindfulness and breath games:** Build emotional regulation
- **Natural remedies:** Like honey for cough (age 1+), or probiotics for tummy health
- **Parent coaching:** Helps reduce stress and improve attachment

Paediatricians are now working alongside child psychologists, Ayurvedic consultants, and even play therapists to offer **gentle, whole-child care.**

"My son used to get ear infections every month. With dietary changes and homoeopathy, he hasn't had one in over a year." – Aditi, parent.

Adolescence: Balancing Body, Brain & Big Feelings

Teen years come with rapid changes and emotional storms. Integrative care provides a safe space for teens to explore their identity while supporting health in body and mind.

Supportive tools for teens:

- **Yoga and movement therapy:** Build confidence and reduce anxiety

- **Art, music, or journaling:** For emotional expression
- **Nutritional counselling:** Helps with hormonal changes, skin health, and mood
- **Stress management:** Teaching breathing, grounding, and screen breaks

Instead of labels or prescriptions alone, integrative care gives teens **skills to cope, grow, and thrive.**

"Mindfulness helped my daughter manage exam stress. She now teaches it to her friends!" – Rahul, father of a 16-year-old

Young Adults: Prevent, Empower, Personalise

This stage is about independence–choosing how you live, eat, move, and care for yourself. It's also when stress, burnout, and lifestyle diseases often start.

What helps?

- **Integrative coaching:** For routines, purpose, and goal-setting
- **Fitness + flexibility plans:** Not just gym workouts–mindful movement
- **Sleep and tech hygiene:** Managing screen time, rest cycles
- **Reproductive health support:** Hormone balance, fertility, menstrual care

With so much life happening online, integrative providers also use **apps and telehealth** to stay connected and offer support.

"I never thought anxiety and digestion were connected—until my naturopath helped me fix both with a few simple changes." – Sneha, 28

Adulthood: Work, Wellness & Wear-and-Tear

Juggling careers, caregiving, and personal health? Welcome to adulthood.

Integrative care steps in to **prevent burnout, support recovery, and promote balance.**

Useful therapies for adults:

- **Acupuncture or cupping:** For back pain, headaches, tension
- **Nutrition + herbs:** To boost energy and immunity
- **Mental wellness:** Through coaching, mindfulness, or therapy
- **Functional medicine testing:** For gut issues, hormone imbalances, fatigue

This stage is where many rediscover traditional medicine—like Ayurveda, TCM, or naturopathy—as part of their healing path.

Fertility, Pregnancy & Postpartum: Wholehearted Support

This chapter of life brings joy, fear, fatigue, and transformation. Integrative care honours all of it.

What's often included:

- **Prenatal yoga & meditation:** Support posture, reduce anxiety
- **Nutrition & herbs:** For iron, folate, and digestive comfort
- **Acupuncture:** For nausea, breech babies, labour prep
- **Postpartum doula support:** For rest, lactation, and emotional balance
- **Ayurvedic or traditional care:** Oil massages, warming foods, body recovery

"After delivery, I felt broken–physically and emotionally. My integrative team helped me rebuild with warmth and wisdom." – Nandini, 34

The Caregiver Years: Holding Others, Caring for Yourself

Whether you're raising children, supporting ageing parents, or both, this phase is often **emotionally taxing.**

Integrative care here focuses on **sustainability**, helping you give without depleting yourself.

What helps:

- Restorative yoga or qigong
- Counselling or caregiver support groups
- Nutrition tweaks to prevent fatigue
- Herbal adaptogens (like Ashwagandha) for stress
- Time in nature, music, or creative expression

When you care for the caregiver, you care for everyone around them, too.

Midlife and Menopause: A Time for Rebalancing

Hormones shift. Energy changes. Priorities realign.

This isn't a "decline"–it's a powerful reset. And integrative therapies help you **move through it with grace.**

Menopause and Midlife Care:

- **Acupuncture or herbs:** For hot flashes, sleep issues, mood
- **Strength-focused movement:** Like Pilates or resistance training
- **Dietary shifts:** Supporting bone, heart, and hormone health
- **Mind-body therapies:** For emotional release and clarity

"I thought I was just moody. Turns out, I needed magnesium, better sleep, and space to breathe." —Jaya, 52

Elder Years: Ageing with Dignity and Comfort

Older adults face changes in mobility, memory, digestion, and independence. Integrative care focuses on **comfort, connection, and quality of life.**

Key supports include:

- **Gentle movement:** Chair yoga, tai chi for balance
- **Music therapy:** For memory, loneliness, mood
- **Massage:** To ease stiffness and improve circulation
- **Herbal remedies:** For sleep, digestion, and joint health
- **Spiritual care:** For meaning, peace, closure

Even in decline, healing is possible—not always curing, but **deep comfort and presence.**

End-of-Life Care: Presence Over Prescription

In the final chapter, integrative medicine offers tools for **peaceful transitions:**

- **Aromatherapy and touch:** For pain and fear
- **Guided imagery or prayer:** For spiritual support
- **Counselling:** For families navigating grief
- **Legacy activities:** Journaling, storytelling, art

The focus here is not just on the patient, but on the **circle of care** that surrounds them.

“Hospice brought a music therapist. My mother sang as she passed. We will never forget it.” – Rina, daughter and caregiver.

The Digital Revolution

Healing is more accessible than ever, thanks to tech:

- Meditation & breathwork apps
- Wearables that track stress & sleep
- Online yoga and qigong classes
- Tele-coaching and digital health logs

Your phone could be your wellness partner.

Summary Snapshot

Life Stage	**Integrative Focus**
Infancy	Bonding, immunity, and sensory development
Childhood	Growth, emotional safety, and allergies
Adolescence	Identity, mood, self-awareness
Young adulthood	Stress, habits, and prevention
Adulthood	Resilience, chronic care, balance
Pregnancy/ Postpartum	Nourishment, recovery, hormones
Midlife/Menopause	Energy, sleep, bone/hormone health
Elderhood	Comfort, mobility, dignity
End-of-life	Spirituality, pain relief, presence

Final Thoughts: Healing at Every Step

Health isn't a fixed destination. It's a **moving rhythm**—changing with your seasons, your age, your needs.

Integrative care respects that. It walks with you, offering tools, compassion, and space to listen to your body at every phase.

So, whether you're caring for a toddler or sitting with an elder...

Whether you're welcoming life or preparing to release it...

There's a healing path waiting to meet you where you are.

Chapter 9:

Policy, Access & The Future Of Integrative Health

Looking Ahead: A Healthcare System That Truly Heals

Imagine a future where your doctor's office includes space for yoga, your health insurance covers acupuncture, and your community clinic offers nutrition coaching and meditation classes.

This isn't a dream. It's already happening–in pockets across the world.

In this final chapter, we examine how policy, access, and innovation are shaping the next generation of integrative care–and how we can make it accessible to all, not just a select few.

Why Policy Matters in Healing

Integrative therapies don't thrive on good vibes alone—they need strong policy support.

When policy changes, more people can:

- Afford care beyond just medications
- Access licensed practitioners in their area
- Choose culturally relevant healing practices
- Be part of a system that treats the whole person

Without policy, integrative care stays niche—available mostly to those with time, money, or awareness.

The Global Movement

Countries around the world are embracing integrative models in exciting ways:

India

- Home to AYUSH (Ayurveda, Yoga, Unani, Siddha, Homoeopathy)
- Integrative clinics blending Ayurveda + allopathy
- Yoga therapy is now part of government health schemes

Germany

- Insurance covers homoeopathy, naturopathy, and more
- Medical schools include integrative medicine training

Brazil

- Offers Reiki, healing circles, and acupuncture in public hospitals
- Strong community-based traditional healing programs

United States

- NIH's NCCIH (National Centre for Complementary and Integrative Health) funds large-scale research
- VA hospitals using acupuncture, meditation, and yoga for veterans

The message? This movement is not fringe—**it's mainstreaming globally,** thanks to supportive policy and public demand.

Insurance & Affordability

Let's face it—integrative care can get expensive if not covered.

But things are changing:

Country	What's Covered
USA	Some plans include acupuncture, chiropractic, and mental health coaching.
UK	GPs prescribe social and nature-based therapies via the NHS.
Germany	Herbal medicine and homoeopathy are reimbursed by insurers.
India	AYUSH hospitals and doctors are integrated into state services

Fair access means **everyone**—not just the wealthy—should benefit from holistic care.

Workforce Training & Recognition

For integrative medicine to grow, we need more:

- **Well-trained practitioners**
- **Cross-disciplinary respect**
- **Licensing and standardisation**

What's helping:

- Medical schools offering integrative medicine fellowships
- Ayurveda and TCM boards developing global standards
- Holistic nursing, coaching, and yoga therapy are gaining recognition

The future? Providers who know both **science and soul**—and are proud to use both.

Digital Health: A Game Changer

The digital era is helping integrative health go global and local:

- **Meditation & sleep apps** (like Insight Timer, Headspace)
- **Telehealth visits** with Ayurveda, nutrition, and mind-body experts
- **Wearables** to track stress, breath, HRV, sleep cycles
- **Online support groups** for chronic illness or healing journeys

The right tech can make healing **personal, portable, and powerful.**

Community & Cultural Healing

True wellness is not isolated. It's communal.

That's why **community-based integrative models** are so powerful:

- Healing circles in tribal and Indigenous communities
- Group yoga or mindfulness in low-income neighbourhoods
- Herbal medicine is taught in community gardens
- Faith-based counselling integrated with mental health services

These models respect tradition, promote equity, and make healing **accessible beyond hospitals.**

Challenges on the Road Ahead

While the vision is bright, the journey has a few bumps:

Challenge	What's Needed
Inconsistent regulations	Clear, global licensing standards
Cost barriers	Insurance reform and public funding
Scepticism	More research, education, and success stories
Urban-rural divide	Mobile care units, digital solutions
Cultural bias	Embracing pluralism in healing systems

"Policy is how we turn possibility into practice." – Public Health Advocate

Future Trends to Watch

1. **Food as medicine** clinics
2. **Integrative oncology** in cancer centres
3. **Green prescriptions** (nature therapy)
4. **Trauma-informed yoga and bodywork**
5. **Personalised herbal protocols** using AI + tradition
6. **Insurance-backed lifestyle medicine coaching**
7. **Cross-trained doctors and healers working together**

These aren't "nice to have." They're **needed** for a healthier, more human future.

Voices from the Field

"Our hospital began using music therapy in palliative care. Families are calling it 'medicine for the soul.'" – Hospital Director, Mumbai

"With online Ayurveda consults, I've helped patients from seven countries in the last year." – Dr. Meenakshi, Integrative Practitioner.

"When the government added yoga to public schools, we saw behavioural improvements across the board." – School Principal, Delhi.

What You Can Do

Change doesn't only come from systems. It starts with people, patients, providers, and communities.

Here's how you can help shape the future:

- Ask for integrative options at your clinic
- Support practitioners who bridge science + tradition
- Vote for policies that expand holistic care
- Share your healing stories–they matter
- Mentor or train in integrative paths
- Start conversations: "What does whole-person care look like here?"

"We are the policy we seek. Every choice we make counts."

Summary Snapshot

Focus Area	Future Direction
Policy	Holistic inclusion in public health systems
Insurance	Covering non-drug therapies and lifestyle care
Workforce	Cross-training and respect for all modalities
Tech	Remote care, wearables, and apps for healing
Community	Grassroots healing spaces and cultural relevance

Final Thoughts: Towards a Future That Heals

Healthcare doesn't have to be cold, clinical, or fragmented. It can be:

- Warm
- Human
- Evidence-informed
- Rooted in both science and wisdom
- Accessible to **everyone**

Integrative health isn't just about better care—it's about **better lives.**

As we look forward, let's keep asking:

"What kind of care would I want for my mother? My child? Myself?"

That's the future we must build.

Conclusion:
A Return To Wholeness

The Journey So Far

You've travelled through a world where healing is more than prescriptions–where food, breath, touch, community, and compassion all have a place.

You've seen how integrative care meets people at every stage of life and in every kind of health journey, with tools that treat not just the body, but the heart and soul as well.

You've met patients, providers, systems, and stories that remind us:

True healing is whole.
True care is personal.
And the future of medicine is already unfolding–
beautifully.

What We've Learned

Let's take a gentle look back at some of the truths this book offered:

- Healing is not just about "fixing" what's wrong–it's about **nurturing what's right**
- Conventional medicine and traditional therapies don't have to compete–they can **cooperate**
- Listening, empathy, and shared decision-making are not extras–they are **essentials**
- Health is not one moment or one measure–it's a **lifelong relationship with your body and mind**

Where Do We Go from Here?

You don't need to memorise every herb or master every breathing technique.

You just need to start somewhere:

- Book that acupuncture session you've been curious about
- Swap one processed snack for something nourishing
- Spend 10 quiet minutes with your breath before bed
- Ask your doctor about integrative options
- Journal about what healing means to you

Small steps. Real care. That's the path forward.

For Practitioners

If you're a provider reading this, thank you.

You're part of the shift. You hold space not just for conditions, but for complexity. And your openness to integrative care makes a world of difference.

Whether you're blending modalities, collaborating with new partners, or simply listening more deeply, you're already practising integrative care.

Keep going.

For Policymakers, Educators, and Leaders

Integrative care belongs not just in private clinics—but in public hospitals, rural centres, and government plans.

The work ahead includes:

- Expanding insurance to cover holistic services
- Training a diverse, cross-disciplinary healthcare workforce
- Funding more community-embedded models
- Honouring local, traditional wisdom as valid and valuable
- Creating a system that uplifts equity, dignity, and access

Healing should never depend on your zip code, income, or background. It should be a **human right.**

Integration in Action: Real Examples

Cancer Care

- **Before:** Chemotherapy only
- **Now:** Chemo + acupuncture, yoga, guided imagery, nutrition counselling

Pain Management

- **Before:** Opioids, surgery
- **Now:** Massage, tai chi, mindfulness, physical therapy, nerve blocks

Mental Health

- **Before:** Medication or talk therapy
- **Now:** Mindfulness-Based Cognitive Therapy (MBCT), breathwork, expressive arts

Patients report better emotional well-being, fewer side effects, and a greater sense of control.

A Closing Reflection

Healing is not always loud or fast. Sometimes it's the quietest thing–the moment someone feels heard, seen, or finally at peace.

It's the patient who learns to breathe through pain.

The elder who finds strength in movement again.

The mother who feels supported—not judged—in her postpartum fog.

The teenager who learns to meditate instead of numbing.

The doctor who says, "Let's try something different—together."

That is integrative care.

That is healing in harmony.

Final Words

Wherever you are—starting your journey, deep in the work, or just curious—know this:

You are not broken.

You are not alone.

You are capable of healing in ways both ancient and new.

This book may end here, but your path is just beginning.

So take what resonates. Leave what doesn't. And keep walking—**with trust, with courage, and with compassion.**

Thank You

Thank you for reading. Thank you for caring. Thank you for believing that a better way is not only possible—but already growing, one heart at a time.

References & Suggested Reading

Global & Policy Perspectives

- **World Health Organisation (2013).** *WHO Traditional Medicine Strategy* 2014–2023.

  A global roadmap illustrating how traditional and integrative therapies are being incorporated into healthcare systems worldwide.

- **National Centre for Complementary and Integrative Health (NCCIH, 2024).** *Complementary, Alternative, or Integrative Health: What's In a Name?*

  A helpful U.S. government guide explaining the terminology and evidence base for integrative practices.

- **Ministry of AYUSH, Government of India (2023).** *AYUSH in Public Health.*

  Outlines how India is blending Ayurveda, Yoga, Unani, Siddha, and Homoeopathy with modern medicine.

Evidence-Based Clinical Research

- Astin, J. A. et al. (2003). *Mind-body medicine: State of the science, implications for practice.*

  Reviews the science behind mind-body practices like meditation, yoga, and relaxation therapies.

- Berman, B. M. et al. (2010). *Acupuncture for chronic low back pain.*

  Landmark study showing acupuncture's role in pain management.

  Strong evidence supports yoga as a complementary therapy for mental health.

- Kligler, B. et al. (2016). *Complementary/integrative therapies that work.*

  A practical review of therapies that have strong scientific backing.

- Langevin, H. M. et al. (2017). *Integrative medicine for pain management.*

  Explains why hospitals and clinics are increasingly turning to integrative pain approaches.

Nutrition & Lifestyle Medicine

- Ornish, D. (2008). *Intensive lifestyle changes and health outcomes.*

  Famous for proving lifestyle changes can reverse heart disease.

- Willett, W. et al. (2019). *Food in the Anthropocene: The EAT-Lancet Commission.*

  Shows how nutrition affects both health and the planet.
- Esch, T. & Stefano, G. B. (2010). The neurobiology of stress management.

  Explains how stress management practices directly affect the nervous system.

Mind-Body & Spiritual Healing

- Kabat-Zinn, J. (1990). *Full Catastrophe Living.*

  A classic introduction to mindfulness and meditation for health.
- Benson, H. (2000). *The Relaxation Response.*

  Explains how relaxation techniques reduce stress and support healing.
- Koenig, H. G. (2012). *Religion, Spirituality, and Health.*

  Explores the role of spirituality and faith in health outcomes.

Integrative Models in Practice

- Snyderman, R. & Weil, A. (2002). *Integrative medicine: Bringing medicine back to its roots.*

  A call to re-centre medicine around the whole person.

- Dodds, S. & Cook, S. (2020). *Integrative care in hospitals.*

  Shows how integrative models are being adopted in real hospital settings.
- Maizes, V., Rakel, D., & Niemiec, C. (2009). *Integrative medicine and patient-centred care.*

  Connects integrative approaches with the growing movement for patient-centred healthcare.

Books & Guides for Deeper Learning

- Weil, A. (2017). *Mind Over Meds.*

  A guide to understanding when drugs are necessary—and when natural healing can work better.
- Khalsa, D. S. (2008). *The Integrative Medicine Approach.*

  A physician's guide to blending conventional and alternative methods.
- Jonas, W. B. & Chez, R. A. (2004). *Toward Optimal Health.*

  Explores prevention and wellness through integrative approaches.

About The Authors

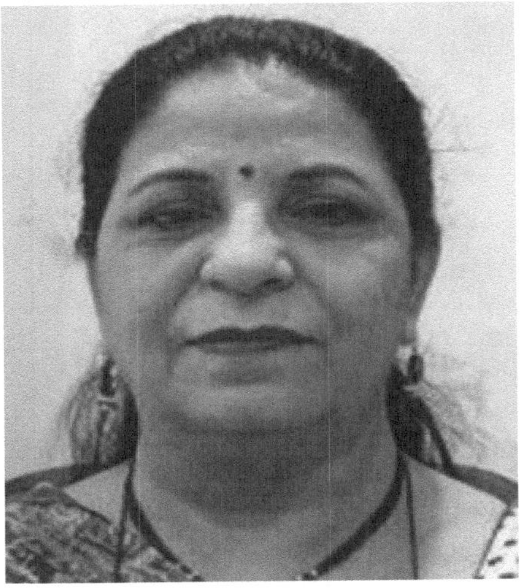

Dr. Jyotika Sharma

Dr. Jyotika Sharma is a respected academician, currently serving as the Head of the Department of Psychology at Sikkim Manipal University, Gangtok, Sikkim, India. With years of experience in research and teaching, Dr. Jyotika has dedicated her career to understanding the intricate connections between the mind and body. Her expertise in psychology and behavioural sciences brings depth and clarity to the emotional and cognitive dimensions of integrative healthcare discussed in this book.

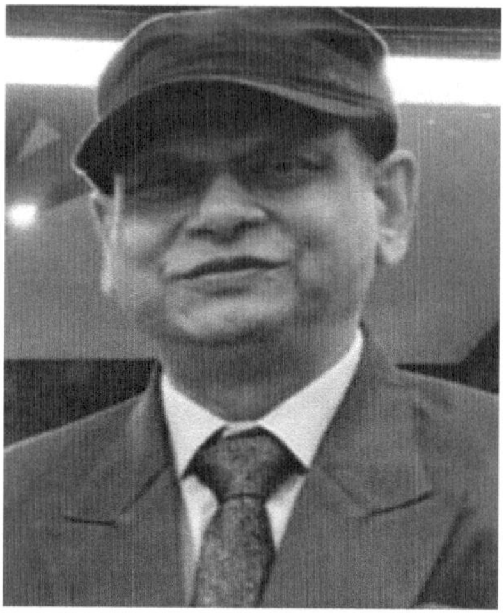

Surajit Debnath

Surajit Debnath brings a unique perspective to this book as a seasoned professional and a lifelong learner. A veteran of the Indian Army, he presently serves as the Head of Engineering Services at Sikkim Manipal University, Gangtok, Sikkim, India. Over the years, Surajit has cultivated a deep interest in holistic health and integrative wellness, inspired by the belief that true well-being lies at the intersection of science, lifestyle, awareness, consistent efforts and emotional balance.

Together, Dr Jyotika and Surajit have combined their diverse expertise to create Healing in Harmony. Their shared vision is simple yet powerful: to inspire readers to explore integrative therapies with curiosity, confidence, and a renewed sense of what it means to heal—completely and harmoniously.